Evidence-Based Practice

A Guide for Nurses

Joan Monchak Lorenz, MSN, RN, PMHCNS-BC
Suzanne C. Beyea, RN, PhD, FAAN
Mary Jo Slattery, RN, MS

D1475175

HCP.

RECEIVED NOV 0 3 2009 MN

Quick-E! Evidence-Based Practice: A Guide for Nurses is published by HCPro, Inc.

HCPro, Inc., provides information resources for the healthcare industry.

HCPro, Inc., is not affiliated in any way with The Joint Commission, which owns the JCAHO and Joint Commission trademarks. MAGNET™, MAGNET RECOGNITION PROGRAM®, and ANCC MAGNET RECOGNITION® are trademarks of the American Nurses Credentialing Center (ANCC). The products and services of HCPro, Inc., and The Greeley Company are neither sponsored nor endorsed by the ANCC. The acronym MRP is not a trademark of HCPro or its parent corporation.

Joan Monchak Lorenz, MSN, RN, PMHCNS-BC, Author

Suzanne C. Beyea, RN, PhD, FAAN, Author

Mary Jo Slattery, RN, MS, Author

Rebecca Hendren, Senior Managing Editor

Emily Sheahan, Group Publisher

Mike Mirabello, Senior Graphic Artist

Amy Cohen, Copyeditor

Adam Carroll, Proofreader

Susan Darbyshire, Art Director

Matt Sharpe, Production Supervisor

Claire Cloutier, Production Manager

Jean St. Pierre, Director of Operations

Advice given is general. Readers should consult professional counsel for specific legal, ethical, or clinical questions.

Arrangements can be made for quantity discounts. For more information, contact:

HCPro, Inc.
P.O. Box 1168
Marblehead, MA 01945
Telephone: 800/650-6787 or 781/639-1872
Fax: 781/639-2982
E-mail: *customerservice@hcpro.com*

Visit HCPro at its World Wide Web sites:

www.hcpro.com and www.hcmarketplace.com

03/2009
21664

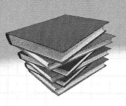

Contents

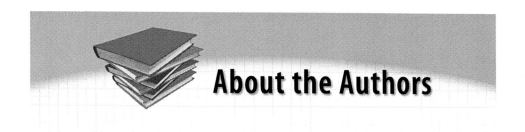

About the Authors

Joan Monchak Lorenz, MSN, RN, PMHCNS-BC

Joan Monchak Lorenz, MSN, RN, PMHCNS-BC, has a varied and well-rounded nursing career in clinical work, consultation and counseling, teaching, and research. She is a clinical nurse educator in the nursing education department at Bay Pines (FL) VA Healthcare System. In this capacity, she works on hospitalwide educational initiatives, provides unit-based programming, and consults with nursing staff on their professional growth. She supports evidence-based practice through her work on the Standards of Care Committee, as past chair of the Evidence-Based Practice Committee, and as past Coordinator of Evidence-Based Practice at Bay Pines.

Lorenz is the founder and president of Clearly Stated, writing and editing health-related material for healthcare professionals and the general public. Her nursing publications include numerous continuing education activities; workshops on a variety of contemporary nursing issues, most recently ones on promoting civility in the workplace; and handbooks on topics such as assessment of the older adult and working with individuals with difficult behaviors.

Lorenz is a graduate of The Johns Hopkins School of Nursing and the Yale University School of Nursing. She is certified as an editor/writer and as an educator by the American Medical Writers Association. She is board-certified by the American Nurses Credentialing Center in psychiatric mental health nursing – adult.

Suzanne C. Beyea, RN, PhD, FAAN

Suzanne C. Beyea, RN, PhD, FAAN, is the director of nursing research at the Dartmouth-Hitchcock Medical Center (DHMC) in Lebanon, NH. Her responsibilities include supporting evidence-based practice, developing the clinical nursing research program for the medical center, and supporting nurses' efforts to use or conduct research. Her activities include providing consultation, education, technical support, and advice related to research, evidence-based practice, and the evaluation of nursing practices and clinical processes. She also serves as the ANCC Magnet Recognition Program® coordinator.

Beyea's nursing publications include journal articles, contributions to textbooks, and monthly columns on research topics and patient safety issues for the *AORN Journal*. She also has numerous publications related to the care of the medical-surgical patient, structured vocabulary, geriatric issues, and patient safety. In addition, she has extensive experience presenting educational sessions related to research, evidence-based practice, best practice, clinical competence, clinical pathways, care of the elderly client, quality improvement and outcomes management, using the clinical value compass to achieve best practices, legal aspects of documentation, and human patient simulation. Currently, she is the primary investigator for an HRSA-funded project called "Nurse Residency Program for Competency Development." She is actively involved in numerous local, regional, and national nursing organizations.

Mary Jo Slattery, RN, MS

Mary Jo Slattery, RN, MS, is the nursing research coordinator at DHMC. She collaborates with the director of nursing research, Suzanne C. Beyea, in the Office of Professional Nursing to support and facilitate research and evidence-based practice efforts in nursing. Her activities include consulting for and assisting with groups and individuals on such topics as online searching, project planning, instrument development, obtaining Institutional Review Board (IRB) approval, data collection, data analysis, and report writing. She manages the departmental review for nursing research studies prior to submission to the IRB, coordinates the use of statistical analysis software, and conducts analysis on selected projects.

Slattery has more than 15 years of experience working with staff nurses in the acute care setting in conducting and using research and, most recently, in evidence-based practice. She is also involved in several professional nursing projects in the institution. She was coprincipal investigator on a DHMC Quality Research Grant–funded project "Evaluation of the Effectiveness of a Targeted Ergonomic Program to Prevent Back and Other Musculoskeletal Injuries in Nursing Personnel." Currently, she is the NDNQI site coordinator and the data manager and analyst on the HRSA-funded project "Nurse Residency Program for Competency Development."

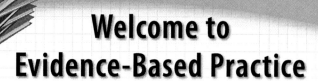

INTRODUCTION

Welcome to Evidence-Based Practice

Nurses often say they don't have time in the day to add more tasks to their already overburdened responsibilities. But incorporating evidence-based practice (EBP) is time well spent, both for nurses' workload efficiency and for the overall care of their patients. As a profession, we must make time for EBP to improve the quality of our care delivery and fulfill our potential as professionals. This book is for nurses who want to understand EBP and grasp the core principles so they can ensure their practice is evidence-based.

You will discover tips and strategies to help you realize better patient outcomes while increasing your knowledge and professional development.

Quick Highlight: Be on the lookout for "quick highlights" that will drive home some of the most crucial points in the book.

We'll take a closer look at:

- Understanding EBP

- Finding sources of evidence

- Critiquing articles to determine validity for your use

- Forming journal clubs and networking with your peers

Let's get started by looking at what EBP really means.

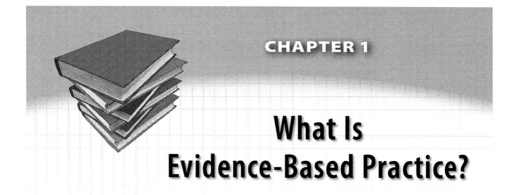

CHAPTER 1

What Is Evidence-Based Practice?

Learning Objectives

After reading this chapter, the learner will be able to:

- Explain evidence-based practice

- Describe how evidence-based practice contributes to improved patient outcomes

The Way We Have Always Done It

Evidence-based practice (EBP) helps nurses provide high-quality patient care based on research and knowledge rather than on traditions, myths, hunches, advice of colleagues, or outdated textbooks. EBP changes the familiar saying "this is the way we have always done it" to "show me the evidence."

EBP is not research; it is the *application* of research to practice. Nursing research adds to the body of nursing knowledge and generates new information. EBP applies that information to your clinical practice.

 Quick Highlight: EBP is the application of research to practice.

Pravikoff, Tanner, & Pierce (2005) report that most nurses provide care in accordance with what they learned in nursing school and rarely use journal articles, research reports, and hospital libraries for reference. That finding, combined with the fact that the average nurse is more than 40 years of age, means many nurses may be providing patient care based on knowledge learned years ago. Practice based on such knowledge does not translate into quality patient care or positive health outcomes. EBP provides a critical strategy to ensure that care is up to date and that it reflects the latest research evidence.

> **Quick Highlight:** EBP is "the conscientious, explicit, and judicious use of the current best evidence in making decisions about the care of individual patients" (Sackett 1998).

The goals of EBP are to:

- Deliver effective nursing care based on the best research and evidence

- Resolve clinical care problems in the clinical setting

- Achieve excellence in care delivery, even exceeding quality assurance standards

- Introduce innovation

(Grinspun, Virani, & Bajnok 2001/2002)

> **Quick Highlight:** Why is EBP important to nursing practice? It:
>
> - Produces better patient outcomes
>
> - Keeps practice current and relevant
>
> - Ensures practice is based on latest research

Nurses use EBP to make their practice more effective. For example, an EBP project reported by Madsen et al. (2005) was undertaken to ascertain the benefits of listening to the bowel sounds of patients who have undergone elective abdominal surgery in determining gastrointestinal (GI) motility. The authors reviewed the literature, conducted an assessment of current practice using the EBP process, and developed and evaluated a new practice guideline for assessing GI functioning after surgery. Through their step-by-step use of the EBP process, they determined that the return of flatus and first postoperative bowel movement were more helpful than listening for bowel sounds in assessing the return of GI motility after abdominal surgery. This evidence-based project resulted in *saving nursing time* with no negative patient outcomes.

Quick Highlight: Blood warmers? Show me the evidence of need!

Nurses can use EBP to make their practice more cost-effective. In an unpublished EBP project at Bay Pines (FL) VA Healthcare System, nurses made a request to the Standards of Care Committee to ask whether blood warmers were needed for each nursing unit that routinely provided blood transfusions to veterans. A group of nurses undertook an EBP project, and after conducting a search of the literature, they recommended the facility follow the guidelines of the ECRI Institute, which states that blood warmers are only needed:

- For massive transfusions (50% of body blood volume)

- When therapy calls for 25% of body blood volume, but the potential exists that more units may be required or that these units may be administered rapidly

- When transfusing blood to patients with cold agglutinins
  (ECRI Institute 2009)

The recommendation was made that blood warmers were not needed on all nursing units that regularly gave blood to veterans. They were only needed in the areas that met the ECRI criteria. This EBP project resulted in *cost saving* for the facility.

Nurses also use EBP to make their practice safer for patients, such as in the example featured on the Web site of the University of Texas Health Science Center at San Antonio's Academic Center for Evidence-Based Practice describing how nurses evaluated the effectiveness of employing two nursing strategies to reduce patient falls and increase patient satisfaction. The nurses' findings indicated that following the implementation of a response to call bell policy and a protocol requiring that the change-of-shift nursing handoff report be given at the patient's bedside, there was a significant decrease in patient falls as well as increased patient satisfaction in the area of promptness of response to call bells and pain control.

The nurses concluded that important patient safety, comfort, and satisfaction outcomes can be improved through the use of innovative evidence-based nursing strategies. These strategies were cost-neutral and had a significant effect on the healthcare experience of hospitalized patients. This EBP project resulted in a *safer, more pleasant environment* for patients.

Quick Highlight: EBP? What's in it for me? It:

- Closes the research-practice gap
- Keeps us current with latest research
- Prevents us from using outdated information

Getting Started

Nurses and other clinicians strive to provide the best care possible, and in today's healthcare environment, evidence-based care is essential. Simply put, using EBP makes sense.

So how do you get started? To fully integrate EBP into your organization and ensure that all nursing practice is based on evidence, you need:

- Administrative support

- Knowledgeable mentors

- Time to complete EBP projects

- Accessible research reports and articles

- Knowledge about the EBP process

Are you ready for the challenge? Although EBP takes commitment and resources, such as time, effort, and dedication, the patient outcomes make it worthwhile. Every patient deserves care that is based on the best current scientific knowledge. Every nurse deserves to work in an environment in which EBP is supported and its results utilized.

Quick Highlight: We ask these questions in EBP:

- What is the clinical practice question?

- What evidence exists that will help answer the question?

- How valid is the evidence?

- How strong is the evidence or results?

- How relevant is it to my practice?

Relationship of Nursing Excellence to EBP

In the past decade, the American Nurses Credentialing Center (ANCC) Magnet Recognition Program® (MRP) has been synonymous with practice environments in which nurses prefer to practice and patients achieve the best outcomes. Evidence exists that hospitals that attract and retain registered nurses demonstrate key characteristics related to their nurse leader, the professional attributes of staff nurses, and their professional practice environment (Scott, Sochalski, & Aiken 1999; McClure & Hinshaw 2002). Additional research supports the benefits of professional practice environments to patients as well as to nursing staff.

The ANCC states that "Evidence-based practice (EBP) is internationally acclaimed as the gold standard for delivering the highest quality care" (2009). It is an essential component of any organization that has achieved MRP status.

You can think about this information when you address the need for EBP support at your facility. EBP's central importance to nursing excellence and its flagship status at any organization deemed worthy of designation means the need for EBP support moves out of the category of "nice to have" and into the category of "need to have."

Quick Highlight: The MRP was developed by the ANCC to recognize healthcare organizations that provide nursing excellence. The program also provides a vehicle for disseminating successful nursing practices and strategies.

Recognizing quality patient care, nursing excellence, and innovations in professional nursing practice, the MRP program provides consumers with the ultimate benchmark to measure the quality of care that they can expect to receive. When *U.S. News & World Report* publishes its annual showcase of America's Best Hospitals, designation as an MRP facility contributes to the total score for quality of inpatient care. Of the hospitals listed on the exclusive 2007 Honor Roll rankings, seven of the top 10 were MRP designated hospitals.

MRP designation is based on quality indicators and standards of nursing practice as defined by the American Nurses Association's *Scope and Standards for Nurse Administrators* (2004). The *Scope and Standards for Nurse Administrators* and other foundational documents form the base upon which the MRP environment is built. The designation process includes the appraisal of qualitative factors in nursing, and these factors, referred to as the 14 Forces of Magnetism, were first identified through research conducted in 1983. The 14 Forces were reconfigured under 5 Model Components in 2008, which places a greater focus on measuring outcomes.

The full expression of MRP designation embodies a professional environment guided by a strong visionary nursing leader who advocates and supports development and excellence in nursing practice. As a natural outcome of this, the program elevates the reputation and standards of the nursing profession.

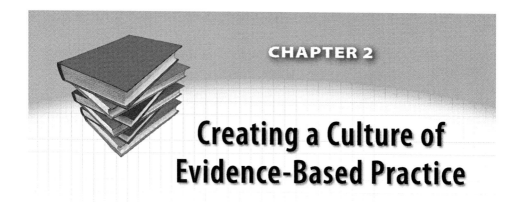

CHAPTER 2

Creating a Culture of Evidence-Based Practice

Learning Objectives

After reading this chapter, the learner will be able to:

- Discuss the resources needed for conducting EBP projects

- Examine strategies for creating a culture of EBP

Getting the Resources You Need

Creating a culture in which everyone can participate in evidence-based practice (EBP) projects requires resources such as subscriptions to electronic journals and databases, access to computers and the Internet, and release time to work on projects and serve on evidence-based councils. Evidence-based projects rarely occur without the combined expertise of a group of clinicians who can readily access the literature and have the time to work on a specific project. Therefore, some first steps to developing an evidence-based culture should be assessing the accessibility of electronic resources and computers and developing a plan to get the resources you need.

Creating a culture of EBP requires administrative buy-in and support. The following are more ways to start incorporating EBP in the nursing practice at your facility. Take some time to evaluate your facility and determine whether these initiatives could be introduced in a timely and effective manner.

Incorporate EBP Concepts into Nursing Practice Committees

Most healthcare facilities have a mechanism for overseeing nursing practice and developing and reviewing nursing policies, procedures, and protocols. One place to start incorporating the practice of EBP is to review your existing nursing committees to determine where the principles of EBP would most likely be best incorporated. The chair of the nursing committee that discusses and implements new nursing policies, protocols, and procedures may be contacted and asked about the use of EBP when reviewing existing standards of nursing practice or implementing new ones. This is often the first and best place to introduce EBP.

Nursing practice leaders need to clearly understand and articulate the benefits of using an evidence-based approach. They need to make sure that every nurse comprehends the need to review the most recently published research findings and not rely solely on personal expertise, opinion, or experience. In this way, best practices can be developed using a knowledge-based rather than an opinion-based approach, and thus evidence-based practices emerge as the organizational standard and expectation. Examining the evidence provides an essential framework for problem-solving and making well-informed decisions.

Opportunities to use EBP exist on all nursing committees that affect practice, whether they are organizationwide or unit-based. EBP is an essential component of every clinical and administrative decision situation. Do not underestimate the importance of answering all questions with evidence.

Quick Highlight: Answer any and all questions with evidence!

Here are some examples of when using EBP is useful:

- When a product purchasing committee is considering adopting a new device, it is important to ask, "What evidence exists that this is a better product?"

- When an administrative team is considering scheduling changes, the group could examine the latest evidence on length of work hours and the relationship to medical errors and patient safety.

- When an infection control committee wants to make a recommendation to change an infection control procedure, they should ask, "What is the evidence for this change?"

Quick Highlight: Make sure every decision made is based on the latest information and uses evidence-based problem-solving approaches.

Regardless of the situation, we need to continually ask ourselves and others difficult questions about why we do what we do.

Quick Highlight: Think about these questions:

- Why do we do it this way?

- Does this practice make sense?

Starting Journal Clubs

Starting a journal club is a great way to read articles that will help update practice. Journal clubs consist of groups of nurses who meet regularly to discuss and critique research articles appearing in scientific journals. Creating one is a good way to get started in evidence-based nursing practice. Journal clubs provide you with the opportunity to learn and develop skills to read and critically evaluate current research to determine how applicable the findings are to your practice area.

The journal club's goals may vary by setting and the expertise of its members. In the beginning, a goal might be to learn how to evaluate research and other EBP articles critically. Later goals may include reading articles to keep up to date with the current research or evaluate current practice based on the research findings in the articles.

An alternative to forming a journal club at your facility is to join an online club that is already established. Some nursing associations and nursing journals offer journal clubs in which a journal article—whether published in that journal or not—is critiqued.

Here are two places you can go to join an online journal club:

- The American Journal of Critical Care (AJCC) features a club called Evidence-Based Review (formerly called the Journal Club). Here you can access the online article, print out a paper copy of the article, respond to the article, read others' responses, or e-mail the article to a colleague. Learn more about AJCC's Evidence-Based Review at *http://ajcc. aacnjournals.org/misc/journalclub.shtml.*

- The Oncology Nursing Forum selects a clinically relevant article and provides specific ideas to facilitate journal club discussion. These questions can be used in a group or alone as a way to keep up to date on current issues. Access the forum online at *www.ons.org/publications/journals/ONF.*

According to Phillips and Glasziou (2004), the most successful journal clubs have a designated facilitator who helps lead the discussion and keeps the group focused. Other roles, which can be rotated among participants, include a journal article presenter and a scribe or reporter to take notes.

Quick Highlight: Start out organized.
When starting a journal club, keep electronic records of the articles read, minutes or discussions of the articles, and any recommendations made. Starting a file system early helps preserve the history of the club and provides access to materials for future reference.

There are many approaches to journal clubs. Identify which format works best for you and your organization. Klapper (2001) recommends having six to 20 regular members, whereas Dyckoff (2004) reports success with inviting all staff nurses in the institution and having about 40 attend each monthly meeting. Some journal clubs meet face to face, whereas others disseminate articles and hold discussion via e-mail. For more information about how to start a journal club and how to critique articles, take a look at Appendix A: Guidelines for Journal Clubs.

Start an EBP Council (or Committee)

Forming an EBP council offers you a forum to discuss areas of interest, a means to coordinate journal clubs, and a place to facilitate educational offerings about EBP and the utilization of nursing research. Members of an EBP council should include nurses from all educational levels who represent clinical departments throughout the organization. Members of the evidence-based council may initially need to energize each other, share their knowledge, and learn together as they investigate all that is involved with introducing EBP to other nurses and to the organization as a whole. One of the council's first learning activities may be to learn how to read and critique research articles or proposals as well as to learn how to use others' EBP projects and undertake EBP projects of its own.

Members of an EBP council may function as facility champions for evidence-based practice. They can focus on activities of concern to all practice settings or develop specialty or topic subgroups to work on specific EBP projects. Setting up the infrastructure for EBP in the facility may also be a major function of the council. Featuring the work of the council through newsletters, posters, nursing grand rounds, and continuing education offerings within the organization helps disseminate information while highlighting the importance of EBP in nursing practice.

Seek Out Mentors

Seeking out mentors with knowledge of EBP to educate, advise, and inspire makes learning about EBP a smoother process. Nurses with graduate degrees and those with advanced practice degrees often take the lead as clinical and organizational experts, coaches, and mentors. Your facility may do well to rely on the experience and expertise of its nurse practitioners and clinical nurse specialists. A nurse prepared as a nurse researcher may also be a great benefit to an organization that is trying to ensure that its nursing practice is evidence-based.

Your facility might want to develop a collaborative relationship with a local school of nursing and/or pursue a joint appointment arrangement, which enables the facility to acquire the services of the school's faculty members, including their expertise in nursing research.

Remember, one of the most critical resources in the EBP process is support from mentors who are experts in the process. If your organization lacks these resources, finding opportunities to collaborate with organizations that have them becomes an essential strategy.

Quick Highlight: Where to go for EBP training.
Here are a few places to check for training opportunities:

- The Academic Center for Evidence-Based Practice at the University of Texas Health Science Center at San Antonio School of Nursing offers a summer institute on EBP: *www.acestar.uthscsa.edu/ default.html*

- The University of Iowa Hospitals & Clinics offers the Advanced Practice Institute: Promoting Adoption of Evidence-Based Practice: *www.uihealthcare.com/depts/nursing/rqom/ evidencebasedpractice/apinstitute.html*

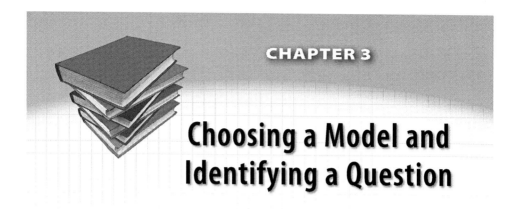

CHAPTER 3

Choosing a Model and Identifying a Question

Learning Objectives

After reading this chapter, the learner will be able to:

- Identify various models of EBP

- Examine how models help structure EBP

- Discuss ways to get started with asking a question

Models of Evidence-Based Nursing Practice

No one model of evidence-based practice (EBP) is a perfect fit for all nursing departments and evidence-based nursing efforts. If your organization does not already have an established nursing EBP group, the first step in choosing a model is to form a representative group of nurses to review and evaluate existing EBP models and determine which would be the best fit for your organization.

Below are a few models that have been described in the literature:

- The Academic Center for Evidence-Based Nursing (ACE) Star Model of Knowledge Transformation®: *www.acestar.uthscsa.edu*

- The University of Colorado's Evidence-Based Multidisciplinary Clinical Practice Model (Goode & Piedalue 1999)

- Rosswurm and Larrabee's Model for Change to Evidence-Based Practice (Rosswurm & Larrabee 1999)

- The Iowa Model of Evidence-Based Practice: *www.uihealthcare.com/ depts/nursing/rqom/evidencebasedpractice/iowamodel.html*

- Johns Hopkins Nursing Evidence-Based Practice Model and Guidelines: *www.nursingknowledge.org/portal/main.aspx?pageid=36&sku=76725*

Iowa Model

The Iowa Model of Evidence-Based Practice (Figure 1) is a well organized and widely used model for EBP. It provides a simple and straightforward framework that most clinicians find easy to follow and fit into their practice environment (Titler et al. 2001).

The Iowa Model of EBP was developed by the Department of Nursing Services and Patient Care at the University of Iowa Hospitals and Clinics in Iowa City to describe knowledge transformation and guide implementation of research into clinical practice. It highlights the importance of considering the entire healthcare system, including the provider, the patient, and the infrastructure.

The steps of the Iowa Model are used to incorporate evidence findings into practice:

- **Step 1:** Identify the trigger. During this step, a problem-focused or knowledge-focused trigger is identified as in need of change. A problem-focused trigger could be a clinical problem or a risk management issue, whereas knowledge triggers might be new research findings or new practice guidelines.

- **Step 2:** Review and critique relevant literature. In this step, you need to check to see whether there is sufficient evidence to make a change in practice.

- **Step 3:** Identify research evidence that supports the change in clinical practice.

- **Step 4:** Implement a change in practice and monitor the outcomes.

Within the model, EBP starts with identifying either knowledge- or problem-focused triggers or need for study. A flow diagram is used to provide a sequential approach and with key decision points, thereby guiding the processes that integrate evidence into practice and help make decisions.

Figure 1 The Iowa Model of Evidence-Based Practice to Promote Quality Care

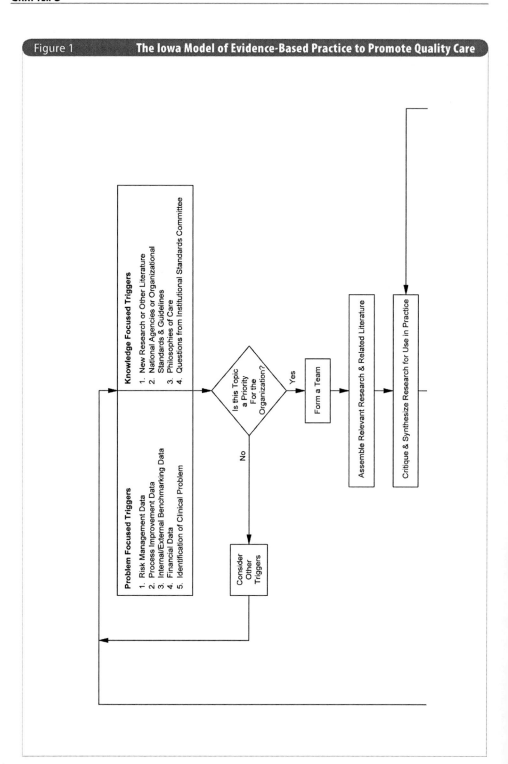

Knowledge Focused Triggers
1. New Research or Other Literature
2. National Agencies or Organizational Standards & Guidelines
3. Philosophies of Care
4. Questions from Institutional Standards Committee

Problem Focused Triggers
1. Risk Management Data
2. Process Improvement Data
3. Internal/External Benchmarking Data
4. Financial Data
5. Identification of Clinical Problem

Is this Topic a Priority For the Organization?

No

Yes

Consider Other Triggers

Form a Team

Assemble Relevant Research & Related Literature

Critique & Synthesize Research for Use in Practice

Quick-E! Pro: Evidence-Based Practice

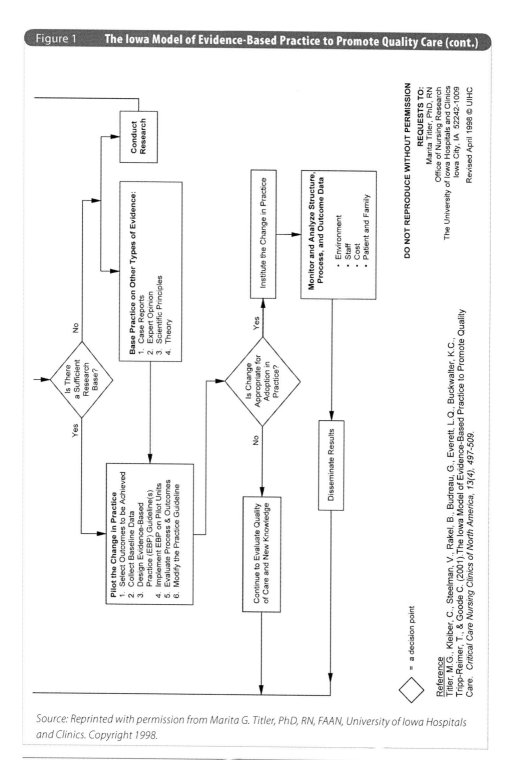

Figure 1   The Iowa Model of Evidence-Based Practice to Promote Quality Care (cont.)

Source: Reprinted with permission from Marita G. Titler, PhD, RN, FAAN, University of Iowa Hospitals and Clinics. Copyright 1998.

Figure 2 is an example of an EBP project using the Iowa Model, as explained in a journal article written by Dontje (2007).

Figure 2	EBP project using Iowa Model
Step and description	**Application/example**
Identify the trigger: either a problem-focused trigger or a knowledge-focused trigger	Knowledge trigger: new guideline related to depression in primary care. Write a clinical question according to the PICO method.
Review and critique relevant literature	In this example, the following databases were used to search for evidence: • Cochrane Library • Clinical Practice Guidelines • Cumulative Index to Nursing and Allied Health Literature • PubMed • U.S. Preventative Services Task Force (USPSTF) guidelines See Chapter 4 for more information about databases and how to access them.
Identify research evidence that supports the change in clinical practice	USPSTF guidelines recommend screening adults for depression in practices where there are systems in place to ensure accurate diagnosis, effective treatment, and follow-up. This guideline is classified as grade B, which indicates that clinicians are strongly recommended to provide the service to eligible patients. More information about grading of guidelines is discussed in Chapter 4.
Implement a change in practice and monitor the outcomes	At a predefined interval (for example, six months to one year) evaluate the change and give feedback to the practice providers on whether the desired outcomes have been reached. This process could coincide with quality improvement activities within the practice.

Source: Dontje, K.J. (2007). "Evidence-Based Practice: Understanding the Process." Topics in Advanced Practice Nursing eJournal 7(4). *Available at* www.medscape.com/viewarticle/567786_print.

ACE Star model

Another model widely used for nursing EBP is the Star Model of Knowledge Transformation®, which is a model for understanding the cycles, nature, and characteristics of knowledge that are used in various aspects of EBP. Known as the ACE Star Model, it is a simple description of the relationships between various stages of knowledge transformation as newly discovered knowledge is moved into practice.

The ACE Star Model places nursing's previous scientific work within the context of EBP, serves as an organizer for examining and applying EBP, and mainstreams nursing into the formal network of EBP.

The following is a brief explanation of each stage of the ACE Star model:

- **Discovery.** Discovery is a knowledge-generating stage. New knowledge is discovered through the traditional research methods. This stage builds the body of research about clinical actions.

- **Evidence summary.** Evidence summary is the first unique step in EBP. The task is to synthesize the information collected during the discovery stage into a single, meaningful statement. This stage is also considered a knowledge-generating stage. A rigorous evidence summary step distinguishes EBP from the old paradigm of research utilization.

- **Translation.** Translation is the stage in which the evidence summaries are transformed into practice recommendations and integrated into practice. This may be the stage where a pilot project is completed.

- **Integration.** Integration is the implementation of innovation into clinical practice. This stage involves changing practices through formal and informal channels, such as revising nursing protocols, policies, or procedures.

■ **Evaluation.** Evaluation is the final stage, and in this stage the outcomes are evaluated. These include evaluation of the effect of the EBP change on patient health outcomes, provider and patient satisfaction, efficacy, efficiency, and economic analysis.

For more information on the ACE star model, visit the Web page of the Academic Center for Evidence-Based Practice at *www.acestar.uthscsa.edu.*

Quick Highlight: The difference between research utilization and EBP. Research utilization is:

- A process of using findings from conducting research to guide practice (Titler, Mentes, Rakel, Abbott, and Baumler 1999).

- The process by which scientifically produced knowledge is transferred to practice (Brown 1999).

EBP represents a broader concept than research utilization. When clinicians use the EBP approach, they go beyond the expertise of clinicians and researchers and consider the patient's preferences and values to guide patient care.

Identifying a Project

Getting started in EBP requires the following:

- Identifying problems, areas of concern, and/or a clinical question

- Prioritizing projects using a system that provides equity and buy-in

- Identifying situations that result in negative or unexpected clinical outcomes or examining hunches made from clinical observations

- Asking questions that are of interest and importance (Beyea 2000).

When considering what kind of EBP project to start with, think about topics that interest you and your fellow nurses, those that are relevant to the specialty or patient population you work with, and ones that can be accomplished in a timely manner. Starting with simple projects first gives the group doing the project time to tease out challenging issues that may arise in completing the process.

To help identify topic areas, look for:

- Nursing activities that you believe are time-wasters or seem futile

- Nursing practices you believe to be based on myth or tradition

- Gaps between something done at your organization and a recently published research article

- Specific nursing techniques or procedures that seem out of date

- Patient problems that are costly or otherwise waste resources

Examples of possible topics include the following:

- How does family presence during CPR affect the process?

- What is the best way to verify placement of nasogastric tubes?

- How best can we prevent ventilator-associated pneumonia?

- What ways have been proven effective in eliminating bloodstream infections related to central lines?

- What are the best practices for oral care for intubated patients?

Begin the process by focusing on solving real-life problems that you or your nursing colleagues come across in your daily work. Making EBP interesting and pertinent to you and your fellow nurses' current practice environment helps ensure everyone's interest, involvement, and commitment to the process.

Focus Your General Question

After identifying your project in general, you need to focus your project, clearly state it, and be able to articulate it to other nurses in a concise manner. There are several methods used to help focus your EBP question. One is called the PICO method. It is important to come up with one method that all nurses working on the project will agree to use. This helps you stay organized and speaking the same language.

Let's use the PICO method to tease out our EBP project question. PICO stands for:

P = Patient population or patient characteristics

I = Intervention or topic of interest being considered

C = Comparison that will be conducted, if any

O = Outcome you are interested in or expect

Example of a PICO question:

Patient characteristics	=	Emotionally ill children
Intervention being considered	=	Limit setting with consequences
Comparison intervention, if any	=	Clear expectations with positive choices
Outcome you're interested in	=	Controlling unwanted behaviors

Now write out the PICO in a question format:

Is limit setting with consequences more effective than clear expectations with positive choices in behaviorally ill children?

Here are some other examples of PICO questions:

- Do children have fewer site reactions when flu vaccine is administered with a 1/2-inch or a 1/4-inch needle?

- Is a visual analogue scale more accurate in assessing dyspnea than asking patients if they are short of breath?

- Do distracters in clinic waiting rooms reduce the dissatisfaction of long waiting times?

- What is the most effective teaching strategy to educate clinical staff on EBP?

- Is a surgical two-minute hand wash as effective as a four-minute hand wash?

Here is another example of a PICO question:

Patient population	=	adult patient – over 18
Interest or intervention	=	screening for Major Depressive Disorder (MDD)
Comparison or control group	=	not screening for MDD
Outcome desired	=	affect provider management

If we write out this question, it becomes: For adult patients older than the age of 18 in primary care settings, does the evidence support whether screening vs. not screening for MDD affects the provider management of individuals with depression?

The PICO framework helps you ask pertinent clinical questions and helps you focus on asking the right questions. It is always important to know exactly what it is that you want to investigate. Having a question that is too broad or vague leads you to become overwhelmed with the amount of information you might uncover.

Quick Highlight: Return on investment.

If your EBP project suggests a practice change, you should also evaluate the return on investment (ROI). ROI is a performance measure used to evaluate the efficiency of a change made (an investment). To calculate ROI, the benefit (return) of an investment is divided by the cost of the investment, and the result is expressed as a percentage or a ratio.

Here is an ROI formula:

$$ROI = \frac{(\text{Gain from investment} - \text{cost of investment})}{\text{Cost of investment}}$$

When thinking about ROI with EBP projects, you can focus on the monetary investment, and sometimes this is important when you are presenting a proposed practice change to hospital administrators. However, other ways to view ROI include:

- Time saving

- Patient satisfaction

- Reduction in complications (these can be quantified into dollar amounts, but we also need to consider the morbidity and suffering of the patient who develops a complication)

- Intangibles such as happier work environment

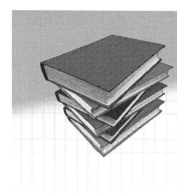

CHAPTER 4

Gathering and Evaluating Evidence

Learning Objectives

After reading the chapter, the participant will be able to:

- Discuss best practices for finding evidence

- Describe how to conduct a literature critique

Finding Evidence

Perhaps one of the biggest challenges in conducting evidence-based practice (EBP) projects is learning how to search the literature, and there are a variety of ways to approach this challenge. Asking a librarian or an educator to come to an EBP council meeting or unit staff meeting to explain how to conduct literature searches gives everyone an overview and understanding of the process. Doing a computer-based real-time search together builds confidence in the process of searching electronic resources and provides you with a real-life learning opportunity.

As the EBP group continues to develop knowledge and awareness, topics for discussion to be addressed include:

- Discerning levels of evidence

- Critiquing research proposals, qualitative research articles, and quantitative research articles

- Understanding reliability and validity

- Formulating an EBP or research question

- Synthesizing the literature

- Developing a clinical practice guideline

Other important areas of study so that you can understand the EBP process and use of research include:

- Overview of models of EBP

- Protection of human subjects

- Ethical issues in nursing research

If your organization has partnered with a local college of nursing, you can take advantage of the facilities at the college. Schedule an appointment with the college reference librarian and ask for an overview of how to access the library's resources. If there is no dedicated medical or nursing library readily available in your area, the local community library may have resources, such as PubMed, that can help you begin to build EBP resources.

If you have the experience or inclination you might want to learn to navigate electronic databases and investigate journals that are available in print or electronic format in your organization. Contact other healthcare facilities in your area and consider visiting one that is doing an EBP project to see what journals and electronic databases they are using.

It is important to find out what your facility offers in the form of online materials and services such as searches. One function of the EBP council might be to compile a list of available journals and databases at your facility and start coordinating educational sessions to promote a better understanding of ways to review the literature. One approach might be to focus the initial EBP committee meetings on education. Emphasizing education about identifying EBP questions, selecting an EBP model, reviewing protocols, and designing studies allows everyone time to develop their skills. This strategy helps you ease into a participatory role as you build your level of understanding and comfort with EBP terms.

Initial topics for the educational sessions could include the following:

- How do I undertake a literature search?

- What is EBP?

- Why is EBP important to me?

- Why is EBP important to my patients and to our organization?

- How do we find time for developing EBP projects?

- How do I get started?

- What resources do I need?

- What resources are available?

Critiquing the Literature

Once you have become comfortable reading and discussing articles you find in your literature searches, then you are ready to start doing formal critiques of the nursing literature. Organize your findings so that you can easily compare and contrast the conclusions or recommendations from the articles. Using a table format to summarize the research articles helps others review the conclusions you reach.

Figure 3 may help to keep you on track.

| Figure 3 | | | Evaluating the strength of the evidence |

Question	Article 1	Article 2	Article 3
Where was the study conducted? What was the setting (e.g., academic medical center, community hospital, rural hospital, or long-term care facility)?			
Who was in the study population? Were study participants similar to patients cared for in your organization?			
How does the study contribute to the body of nursing knowledge? Do the study findings make sense?			
What are the implications for nursing practice/education/research?			
What additional questions does the study raise?			
Does the empirical evidence presented in this article support a change in practice?			
What resources would be required to implement the change?			
Would the benefits of this practice change or outweigh the risks to patients?			
What will be the outcome of this practice change on nurses, patients, or the organization?			
How will the practice change be evaluated?			

Evaluating Web Sites

Not all Web sites are created equal. Nurses need a discerning eye to make sure that the Web sites used for finding literature are reputable. Look for evidence that the Web site is monitored and evaluated by experts. Look for Web sites that are run by a respected real-life person, organization, or institution in which you already have confidence. When you're on a Web site, click on its "About us" page to find out more about who runs the site.

Most reputable Web sites are run by:

- Federal government agencies

- Universities

- Medical associations

- Reputable healthcare-related organizations

Less reputable Web sites (in terms of literature findings) are those run by companies trying to sell products and services, bulletin board sites (where anyone can post his or her opinion), and personal Web sites. Look for these symbols to show whether a Web site has been approved by an independent accreditation group:

- The Health on the Net (HON) code is given by the Health On the Net Foundation to Web sites that provide useful and reliable online medical and health information.

- A URAC code is given by the Utilization Review Accreditation Commission, which is an independent nonprofit organization well known as a leader in promoting healthcare quality through its accreditation and certification programs.

Quick Highlight: To learn more about how HON and URAC work, visit their Web sites:

- *www.hon.ch*

- *www.urac.org*

Other resources exist that are helpful when you are trying to evaluate health-care information found on the Internet. Here are some sites that might be helpful in guiding you in the evaluation process:

- Johns Hopkins Library *(www.library.jhu.edu/researchhelp/general/evaluating)*

- University of California Berkeley Library *(www.lib.berkeley.edu/TeachingLib/Guides/Internet/Evaluate.html)*

- Cornell Library *(www.library.cornell.edu/olinuris/ref/research/skill26.htm)*

One of the biggest challenges of evaluating evidence is learning how to critique the literature. You might ask a nurse researcher or PhD nurse at your facility to provide educational sessions. Initial topics for the educational sessions could include the following:

- How do I critique an article?

- Who is available to help?

- What resources are available?

- How are resources accessed, and what support is available for their use?

Tool for Evaluating Web Sites

When examining Web pages and the content within these resources, one way to avoid taking Web resources at face value is to look for the primary source of the evidence and evaluate how conclusions were reached. Conduct a systematic evaluation of the information's worth. A simple mnemonic that can be used to evaluate Web sites is, "Are you PLEASED with this site?" Figure 4 explains how to use this tool.

Figure 4		Are you PLEASED with this site?
	Definition	**Action to be taken**
P	Purpose of the site	Determine whether the purpose is clearly explained and whether it fits the content on the site.
L	Links	Determine whether the links are current and whether they link to reputable sources.
E	Editorial	Determine whether the content is up to date and correct.
A	Author	Identify the author and his or her credentials for providing the presented information.
S	Site	When reviewing the site, evaluate its ease of use and how the content is presented.
E	Ethical	Consider whether contact information for the author is readily available and whether appropriate disclosures about the content are provided.
D	Dates	Ask when the information was posted and whether the Web site has been recently reviewed and updated.

Source: Nicoll and Beyea 2000.

Take a look at the end of this book for Appendix B, which provides a checklist of questions to ask when evaluating Internet resources.

Assessing the Strength of the Evidence

Several rating systems have been developed to help judge the strength of the evidence available about a particular topic. These levels of the strength of evidence become very important when reviewing or developing clinical practice guidelines. Such classification systems help clinicians and others rate the quality and rigor of the literature. In the United States, various organizations rate the strength of evidence and use different methods. For example, the Agency for Healthcare Research and Quality (AHRQ)—whose mission is "to improve the quality, safety, efficiency, and effectiveness of health care for all Americans"—is a recognized authority on rating scientific evidence.

AHRQ's rating scale includes five categories for rating evidence, arranged from the strongest to the weakest. See Figure 5 for the rating scale.

Figure 5	Agency for Healthcare Research and Quality (AHRQ) rating scale
Classifications	**AHRQ strength of evidence**
1A	Meta-analysis of multiple well-designed controlled studies
1	Well-designed randomized controlled trials
2	Well-designed nonrandomized controlled trial (quasi-experiments)
3	Observational studies with controls (retrospective studies, interrupted time studies, case-control studies, cohort studies, with controls)
4	Observational studies without controls (cohort studies without controls and case series)

Another system for rating the strength of evidence comes from the U.S. Preventive Services Task Force (USPSTF), which grades the quality of the overall evidence for a particular service using a five-category system. This system also makes suggestions for practice. Take a look at Figure 6 for an overview of the USPSTF system.

Figure 6		**USPSTF grading system**

Grade	Definition	Suggestions for practice
A	The USPSTF recommends the service. There is high certainty that the net benefit is substantial.	Offer/provide this service.
B	The USPSTF recommends the service. There is high certainty that the net benefit is moderate or there is moderate certainty that the net benefit is moderate to substantial.	Offer/provide this service.
C	The USPSTF recommends against routinely providing the service. There may be considerations that support providing the service to an individual patient. There is at least moderate certainty that the net benefit is small.	Offer/provide this service only if other considerations support offering or providing the service to an individual patient.
D	The USPSTF recommends against the service. There is moderate or high certainty that the service has no net benefit or that the harms outweigh the benefits.	Discourage the use of this service.
I Statement	The USPSTF concludes that the current evidence is insufficient to assess the balance of benefits and harms of the service. Evidence is lacking, of poor quality, or conflicting, and the balance of benefits and harm cannot be determined.	Read the clinical considerations section of the USPSTF Recommendation Statement. If the service is offered, patients should understand the uncertainty about the balance of benefits and harms.

In addition to the grading and suggestions for practice table, the USPSTF also offers a level of certainty regarding net benefit tool to use with particular practices. The USPSTF defines "certainty" as "likelihood that the USPSTF assessment of the net benefit of a preventive service is correct." The net benefit is defined as benefit minus harm of the preventive service as implemented in a general, primary care population. The USPSTF assigns a certainty level based on the nature of the overall evidence available to assess the net benefit of a preventive service.

Figure 7 is an example of how the USPSTF rates evidence, from a high level of certainty to a low level of certainty.

Figure 7	Level of certainty

Level of certainty	Description
High	The available evidence usually includes consistent results from well-designed, well-conducted studies in representative primary care populations. These studies assess the effects of the preventive service on health outcomes. This conclusion is therefore unlikely to be strongly affected by the results of future studies.
Moderate	The available evidence is sufficient to determine the effects of the preventive service on health outcomes, but confidence in the estimate is constrained by such factors as: • The number, size, or quality of individual studies • Inconsistency of findings across individual studies • Limited generalizability of findings to routine primary care practice • Lack of coherence in the chain of evidence As more information becomes available, the magnitude or direction of the observed effect could change, and this change may be large enough to alter the conclusion.
Low	The available evidence is insufficient to assess effects on health outcomes. Evidence is insufficient because of: • The limited number or size of studies • Important flaws in study design or methods • Inconsistency of findings across individual studies • Gaps in the chain of evidence • Findings not generalizable to routine primary care practice • Lack of information on important health outcomes More information may allow estimation of effects on health outcomes.

Source: U.S. Preventive Services Task Force ratings. Available at www.ahrq.gov/clinic/uspstf07/ratingsv2.htm.

Putting Research into Action

Once you have developed your EBP question, searched the literature, and determined the strength of the evidence, you should evaluate whether the changes work. When deciding to make EBP changes, always evaluate the outcomes of any changes. Never assume that changes in clinical practice will have the anticipated outcomes. Therefore, pilot-test the changes on one or two clinical units to help detect unexpected outcomes and to understand any implementation-related problems. Based on the findings from the pilot units, you can decide to move forward with the practice change in all of the applicable units or to modify or reject the change.

After you have instituted a practice change based on the best evidence, re-member that ongoing monitoring is important. Set up a process to continue to monitor the change at specific intervals of time, evaluate the findings, and determine whether the change has sustained value over the long term. Even if the implementation is successful at the outset, the project is not completed because it is not known whether the success will continue over time. Any evidence-based project requires clinicians to monitor the findings in an ongoing fashion. New knowledge or information may be developed and will need to be integrated into the practice change.

Quick Highlight: Evidence-based projects are never complete; they require the ongoing efforts of dedicated professionals who are willing to question their practice and continually find ways to improve patient outcomes.

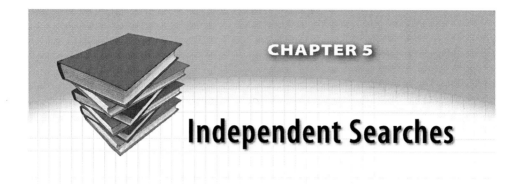

CHAPTER 5

Independent Searches

Learning Objectives

After reading this chapter, the participant will be able to:

- List online sources for evidence

- Evaluate various online sources of evidence

Many resources are readily accessible with the click of a computer mouse. This chapter provides guidance on how to access resources online. Although you might be tempted to Google your evidence-based practice (EBP) focus question, using reputable professional healthcare Web sites is best.

But then again, sometimes using Google gives you a place to get started and often leads to other sites that are more scientific. So if you use Google or other search engines, be sure to use them with caution.

A few of the many helpful Internet resources for EBP include the National Library of Medicine, the Cochrane Library of Databases, the National Guideline Clearinghouse, the Joanna Briggs Institute, and Netting the Evidence.

Learning more about each of these resources and others listed in this chapter serves as an important first step to EBP. The materials available on each of these sites provide a beginning understanding of many of the resources clinicians can access when undertaking evidence-based projects. Many of these Web sites provide links to resources that also may be helpful. It is wise to check back on these Web sites periodically as they update their information, which affords you the opportunity to stay current in your knowledge about EBP.

National Library of Medicine

The National Library of Medicine (NLM) *(www.nlm.nih.gov)* serves as a key resource for many databases in addition to those on Medline. This is a good place to start your search for evidence as the databases included on the NLM Web site may be pertinent to various evidence-based projects.

Resources available through the NLM include MedlinePlus, ClinicalTrials.gov, NIHSeniorHealth, ToxTown, Household Products, Genetics Home Reference, and AIDSinfo. Each of these databases includes topic-specific information that may relate to focused evidence-based projects. For example, perhaps you are seeking information about the effect of a certain healthcare concern for AIDS patients. A key resource in that effort might be the NLM's AIDSinfo, which offers current information on clinical trials for AIDS patients and federally approved HIV treatment and prevention guidelines.

Cochrane Library

A popular resource for organized reports on EBP is the Cochrane Database of Systematic Reviews, which provides systematic reviews that reflect the best available information about healthcare interventions and their effectiveness. Expert teams complete comprehensive literature and research reviews, evaluate the research, and present integrated summaries of the best evidence. These reviews are updated regularly and incorporate new research findings when they become available. The abstracts of the various reviews are available free of charge on the Cochrane Library Web site *(www.cochrane.org/reviews/ clibintro.htm)* and provide a valuable source of healthcare information. In some instances, plain-language summaries are provided using a minimum of technical terms. Many biomedical libraries give users access to some or all of these databases.

Quick Highlight: The Cochrane Collaboration's Web site contains a wealth of extremely useful information:

- For free informational brochures, visit *www.cochrane.org/resources/ brochure.htm*

- For free access to the Cochrane Reviewer's Handbook, visit *www. cochrane.org/resources/handbook/index.htm*

Note: Some of the Cochrane Library databases are indexed in the Cumulative Index to Nursing and Allied Health Literature (CINAHL).

The Cochrane Library includes the following databases:

- Cochrane Database of Systematic Reviews

- Database of Abstracts of Reviews of Effects

- Cochrane Controlled Trials Register

- Cochrane Methodology Register

- NHS Economic Evaluation Database

- Health Technology Assessment Database

- Cochrane Database of Methodology Reviews

National Guideline Clearinghouse

The Agency for Healthcare Research and Quality (AHRQ), in partnership with the American Association of Health Plans and the AMA, sponsors the National Guideline Clearinghouse (NGC). The NGC *(www.guideline.gov)* provides a virtual resource for evidence-based protocols. Protocols and guidelines on this Web site are developed by teams of experts who have reviewed and synthesized the literature and rated the strength of the research findings, thus providing clinicians—as well as patients and healthcare consumers—with guidance about best practices for a particular condition. This searchable Web site allows users to search by disease or condition, measures or tools, and the developing organization; it also includes review guidelines that are in progress or those that have been archived.

Joanna Briggs Institute

The Joanna Briggs Institute *(www.joannabriggs.edu.au)* is an international nonprofit research and development organization specializing in evidence-based resources for healthcare professionals in nursing, midwifery, medicine, and allied health. It supports a "collaborative approach to the evaluation of evidence from a diverse range of sources, including experience, expertise, and all forms of vigorous research" and the implementation of the best available evidence. The institute brings together practice-oriented research activities to improve effectiveness, processes, and outcomes. Included among some of its activities are:

- Conducting systematic reviews of the research

- Collaborating with expert researchers and clinicians to develop best practices

- Offering courses in evidence-based nursing

- Performing primary research, when indicated by the systematic review findings

- Promoting cost-effective, evidence-based nursing

- Planning and organizing research colloquia

The Joanna Briggs Institute Web site also provides comprehensive nursing resources and opportunities to collaborate with others interested in similar efforts and projects.

Netting the Evidence

Another helpful resource is Netting the Evidence *(www.shef.ac.uk/scharr/ir/ netting)*. This Web site provides a searchable database for finding evidence for practice. Users can find quick links to various Internet resources to answer statistical questions, guide bedside diagnosis, access EBP guideline databases, and explore a wide variety of other evidence-based resources. This searchable database is intended to facilitate evidence-based healthcare by providing support and access to useful learning resources, including an evidence-based virtual library, software, and journals.

Task Force on Community Preventive Services

The Task Force on Community Preventive Services *(www.thecommunityguide. org)* is an independent, nonfederal task force consisting of 15 members, including a chair, appointed by the director of the Centers for Disease Control and Prevention. The task force's membership is multidisciplinary and includes representatives from state and local health departments, managed care, academia, behavioral and social sciences, communications sciences, mental health, epidemiology, quantitative policy analysis, decision and cost-effectiveness analysis, information systems, primary care, and management and policy.

U.S. Preventive Services Task Force

The U.S. Preventive Services Task Force *(www.ahrq.gov/clinic/uspstfab.htm)* was convened by the U.S. Public Health Service in 1984 to systematically review the evidence regarding the effectiveness of a wide range of clinical preventive services, including screening tests, counseling, immunizations, and chemoprophylaxis. The task force publishes the Guide to Clinical Preventive Services and is closely affiliated with AHRQ.

Veterans Evidence-Based Research Dissemination Implementation Center

Veterans Evidence-Based Research Dissemination Implementation Center's (VERDICT) *(www.verdict.research.va.gov)* mission is to foster a knowledge-based healthcare system in which clinical, managerial, and policy decisions are based upon sound information from research findings. The multidisciplinary team addresses systematic implementation of evidence in clinical practice within the Veterans Health Administration, leading to integrated models of care and improved service, quality, and efficiency. Learning resources available include VERDICT Briefs.

Centre for Evidence-Based Medicine University Health Network

Some electronic resources may be helpful to you or your facility's evidence-based councils in their efforts to develop knowledge and skills when embarking on the EBP journey. For example, the Centre for Evidence-Based Medicine University Health Network *(www.library.utoronto.ca/medicine/ebm)* provides numerous resources to help develop, disseminate, and evaluate resources for teaching and practicing evidence-based medicine. The headings on its home page include an introduction to evidence-based medicine, syllabi for practicing evidence-based medicine, evidence resources, a glossary, and many other resources.

Centre for Health Evidence

Another Web site that might be helpful in developing EBP expertise is the Canadian Centre for Health Evidence *(www.cche.net)*. This resource intends to help patients, clinicians, and policymakers by providing resources and helping people acquire, appraise, and use knowledge and develop an understanding of how the information is utilized. One of the many helpful resources on this site includes numerous articles on EBP that are available in a downloadable format. These articles would be especially helpful to any organization that lacks electronic library resources.

Other Web Resources

Numerous other nursing-specific, evidence-based Web resources have been developed, including the following:

- University of Minnesota *(http://evidence.ahc.umn.edu/ebn.htm)*

- McGill University Health Centre's Research & Clinical Resources for Evidence Based Nursing *(www.muhc-ebn.mcgill.ca)*

The Web sites and lists provided in this chapter are not a comprehensive listing resource, but they provide a beginning point if you want to learn more. Entering the terms "evidence-based practice and nursing" in a search engine such as Google can result in other resources as well. One of the advantages of using some of the Web sites listed in this chapter is that they limit the hits you will receive to those that have scientific merit. If you use Google to search for a certain healthcare concern or condition, such as diabetes mellitus, you might obtain millions of possible links. The links provided by the sites listed here narrow your initial search and, in addition, offer some opportunities to learn the basics of EBP while exploring them.

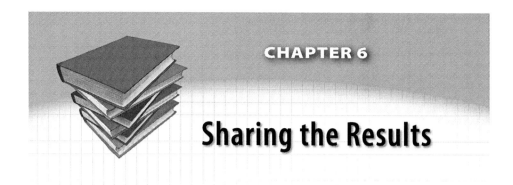

CHAPTER 6

Sharing the Results

Learning Objectives

After reading this chapter, the learner will be able to:

■ Discuss best practices for disseminating EBP information

Ways to Publicize EBP Projects

The final and often most important part of completing evidence-based practice (EBP) projects is to share what you have learned with others. Disseminating and publicizing the results of EBP projects supports the culture of EBP. It serves a critical role in advancing nursing and increasing staff nurse involvement in nursing research efforts. Enabling nurses to understand the importance of contributing to nursing science helps them understand the importance of their work and its value to patients and the larger nursing community.

There are many ways to spread the word about the great work you and your nurse colleagues have done with your EBP projects. Some hospitals have a nursing EBP project day during which certain projects are presented as papers and others are offered in a poster format. Other ways to share your EBP work include:

- EBP bulletin boards on the nursing unit with holders for handouts

- EBP corner on each clinical unit—this corner may be a shelf or table within each unit's break room where articles, newsletters, and other materials can be distributed

- Distribution of EBP minutes via e-mail, hard copy, or on an EBP board/corner

- Access to an EBP hotline that provides information regarding evidence-based questions or concerns

- Placement of posters in high-traffic areas, such as where staff nurses eat lunch, to increase the chances that they will be read

- EBP games, such as a crossword puzzle or bingo, to encourage participation, with small prizes, candy, or handouts as incentives

Publish an EBP Newsletter

Try using an EBP newsletter to distribute highlights from your EBP council meeting minutes and to disseminate other EBP updates. It could include some of the following headings:

- EBP online resources and how to access these resources

- Examples of EBP

- EBP term of the month

- Update from the evidence-based nursing council and meeting dates/times

- Overview of EBP initiatives within your organizations

- Facilitators and barriers of EBP

Spread the Word Outside Your Facility

Don't be shy. To gain a broader audience for the work you and your colleagues have done with EBP at your facility, share what you have learned by participating in poster or oral presentations at local, regional, national, or even international conferences. If you have never submitted an abstract for presentation at a nursing conference, ask for help from someone who has. The most important thing to remember when submitting materials for acceptance at nursing events is to follow the directions given and make sure that you include everything asked for in the proper format. Sending in a submission that is longer than requested or not in the format requested is almost surely going to be rejected.

In addition to presentations of your work at nursing events, think about publishing your work in nursing journals. Each nursing journal has requirements and guidelines for submission. Again, make sure you follow these guidelines to ensure that your submission is taken seriously. Make sure that you submit your ideas to a journal that will be likely to publish your article (i.e., one that has published similar articles on similar topics in the past). One way to look for a journal that might publish your work is to look through the table of contents of the most recent issues of the journal to see what type of articles it has published recently.

It is also important to note that you do not have to publish your work in a peer-reviewed publication. If the purpose of your article is to share information, then consider that non–peer-reviewed nursing publications often have a wider audience than reviewed journals. So include these publications in your requests, and be sure to follow their guidelines for submission as well.

Another way to test the waters to see whether there is interest for your work is to send a query e-mail to the editor, briefly describing your project and asking whether it is something the journal would be interested in pursuing for publication. You can obtain the e-mail addresses of journal editors from the journal's Web page.

> **Quick Highlight:** Where can I find a list of nursing journals?
> Check out these Web sites for lists of nursing journals and search for each by title:
>
> - NursingCenter.com
>
> - CINAHL® (the Cumulative Index to Nursing and Allied Health Literature) has a listing of core nursing journals covered in its database: *www.cinahl.com*

Finding a strategy for sharing information about your EBP work that is consistent with organizational culture and that will grab staff nurses' attention will prove most helpful. Be creative and try to connect with as many potentially interested staff nurses as possible to build enthusiasm for EBP.

> **Quick Highlight:**
> Here's a quick summary of everything you have just covered and the steps you must follow in the EBP process:
>
> 1. Formulate a clinical question
>
> 2. Search the literature
>
> 3. Read and evaluate the literature
>
> 4. Make a decision based on the literature
>
> 5. Apply what you found to your practice
>
> 6. Evaluate the results and whether the change resulted in improvements.
>
> 7. Tell others what you found and how it worked

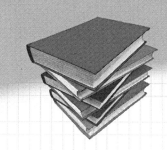

Guidelines for Journal Clubs

1. Recruit members: Place notices on bulletin boards or electronic lists.

2. Seek the support of nursing leadership from the beginning so that organizational issues will be easier to address later on.

3. Set meeting schedules ahead of time and at times of best staff availability. Lunchtime or change of shift are two logical options, but also consider the night shift. Determine meeting frequency by each particular setting.

4. Choose a convenient meeting location.

5. Identify journal articles for discussion. Availability of electronic databases makes literature searches easy to perform if the resources are available for access within your organization.

6. Select topics that are clinically relevant to you and the other members of the group. Journal clubs work best if you identify topics that are relevant to your practice setting.

7. Distribute copies of the selected article and any critique guidelines in advance to allow enough time for everyone to read them before the scheduled meeting. In organizations with electronic library resources, the article link may be e-mailed to participants.

8. Invite other members of the healthcare team to your journal club. The club can be interdisciplinary as long as it focuses on nursing practice.

9. Have fun and encourage all to participate.

10. At the end of each session, evaluate the journal club and select a topic for the next meeting.

Learning How to Critique the Nursing Literature

Once a journal club is formed, you may wonder how to choose an appropriate article and how to go about critiquing one.

The first step is to select articles that are research-based and from a peer-reviewed journal. Other guidelines for selecting appropriate research or EBP articles are:

- Choose a current article. Articles should be no more than five years old.

- Studies from medical journals should be limited and used only if the topic relates to a nursing issue. Be sure the article focuses on nursing interventions, not medical interventions.

- Either quantitative or qualitative research articles are appropriate for review (see Appendix C for explanations of quantitative and qualitative research).

- Use of secondary sources or nursing textbooks must be avoided.

- When possible, select articles with a comparable patient population to the population you serve.

If you are just starting your journal club, make sure the articles selected are appropriate for nurses who are in the novice to advanced beginner stage of EBP knowledge development. Nurses learn the EBP process and how to critique research studies in stages. Initially, select research studies that do not bog down the group in complex statistical tests. If the article does have complex statistics, seek additional guidance with that aspect of the review if it is beyond the scope of the facilitator. The critique and discussion will be much more meaningful if the article selected is relevant to the group and addresses a current clinical problem.

Guidelines for the Critique of Nursing Research Articles

The overall goal of a nursing research article critique is to evaluate a study's merits and its applicability to clinical practice. A research critique goes beyond a review or summary of a study; it carefully appraises a study's strengths and limitations. By evaluating a study's components, you can objectively assess a study's validity and significance.

Several guidelines for the appraisal of evidence have been published in print and online. In addition to nursing research textbooks, several published guidelines for how to review single research studies can help you in your journal club endeavors.

The following resources specifically target the critical appraisal of research studies:

- Critical appraisal worksheets in the EBM Toolbox, Center for Evidence-Based Medicine at Oxford *(www.cebm.net)*.

- Users' Guide to Evidence-Based Practice. Site maintained by the Canadian Centre for Health Evidence *(www.cche.net/usersguides/ start.asp)*. (Originally published in the *Journal of the American Medical Association.*)

Beyea and Nicoll (1997) published a simple guide of 10 questions to use when reading and discussing a research article. Use it to assess the quality of the study and to determine its applicability to clinical practice. This tool is an effective introduction to critiquing and is especially helpful to the novice consumer of research. (See Figure A.)

Figure A	Ten questions for a research report review

10 questions for critiquing	Clarifying points
1. What is the research question?	Is it understandable? Can you paraphrase it?
2. What is the basis for this research question?	To what aspect of nursing practice, education, or theory does it relate?
3. Why is this research question important?	Is it clinically relevant?
4. How was the research question studied?	What methods were used?
5. Does the study make sense?	Does the method used match the research question?
6. Were the correct subjects selected for the study?	How were they selected? Did they obtain informed consent?
7. Was the research question answered?	Describe the findings.
8. Does the answer make sense?	Do the findings support the hypothesis?
9. What is next?	Research leaves many unanswered questions. What would be the next question to explore?
10. So what?	Is this study and its findings relevant to clinical practice?

Source: Beyea, S.C., and Nicoll, L.H. (1997). Ten questions that will get you through any research report. AORN Journal 65 (5): 978–979.

With experience, educational sessions, and mentoring, your knowledge and confidence levels will continue to increase. EBP, like any new skill, takes practice. Journal clubs are a great way to learn the skills necessary to evaluate the evidence and decide whether it's applicable to specific practice areas.

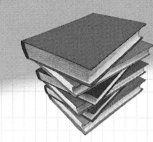

Process for Evaluating Internet Sources

1. Who is the author, and are his or her credentials listed? Is there an e-mail address or a way of contacting the author if questions arise? Is the researcher the person who is responsible for the creation of the site?

2. When determining accuracy, are references listed? Does the article seem credible? Is the article based on information that the reader already knows to be true? Is statistical data listed and, if so, is it presented in graphs or tables for clear understanding?

3. Is the document current? When was the site created? Is there any indication that the information is updated or revised frequently? Are there links to other Web sites and are these current?

4. Is the Web page free of advertising? If advertising is present, is it separated from the written material? Is the information objective and free from author bias? Does it include provocative language?

5. What is the URL of the document? Does it reside on the Web server of an organization that may have extreme points of view?

6. Does the page appear to be complete, or are there references to additional sources that complete the information presented?

7. What is the main purpose of the page? Is the emphasis of the page technical, scholarly, popular, or other?

8. Is the page easy to use, or does it require special software? If the latter is true, can the software be downloaded free of cost? Is the site open to anyone with access to the Internet?

Source: Flaugher, M. (2008). Nursing Research Program Builder: Strategies to Translate Findings into Practice. *Marblehead, MA: HCPro, Inc.*

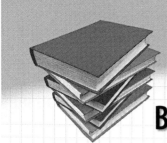

Basic Research Designs

Research design falls into two major categories: quantitative and qualitative. Quantitative research is defined as measurable data, whereas qualitative research is not measurable, but examines a subject's values and beliefs on a specific concept that is being examined. These values are then categorized into similar themes and conclude with a narrative summary by the researcher.

Major differences between the two types of research design include sampling procedures and findings. In quantitative studies, samples are selected that will be representative of the population before data are collected. In qualitative studies, subjects are chosen who are currently experiencing or who have experienced the concept being studied. Findings in quantitative studies are based on the research question and differences in treatment or relationships to the factors being studied. The findings lend themselves to statistical testing, with specific numbers assigned to support or not support the results.

An example of a quantitative clinical study question could be: What differences exist among geriatric-based nurses from an inpatient setting versus a nursing home setting on perceptions and knowledge of chronic elderly pain management? The two groups (inpatient and nursing home) might be given a questionnaire regarding perceptions and knowledge. Results could show the mean average score within the two groups, and if educational level and time in practice were also obtained, a correlational study (Pearson) could be used to determine whether these factors had an influence on knowledge.

An example of qualitative research could include a small group of elderly patients with documented chronic pain. These subjects could be interviewed using a selected number of specified questions regarding how pain interferes with their quality of life. No statistical testing would be used, but common themes or findings could be ascertained and a summary of findings could be extrapolated.

Within quantitative and qualitative research, design can also be narrowed down under further categories:

- **Historical:** Collection of data from different sources of events that have already occurred

- **Case studies:** In-depth review that helps gain insight from natural observations to provide additional information

- **Surveys:** Collection of data from specific populations on a limited topic

- **Experimental:** Manipulation of one or more independent variables and observation of the effect on the dependent variable

- **Quasi-experimental**: Experimental study lacking randomization

- **Ex post facto:** Collection and study of data on a topic that has already occurred

- **Methodological:** Studies that develop or evaluate research tools or techniques

- **Observational:** Monitoring of subjects in public places with or without manipulation of the environment

- **Epidemiological:** Identification of risk factors for a particular condition

- **Prospective:** Observation of events and responses after subjects have been identified

- **Longitudinal:** Examination of one or more groups over an extended period of specified time

- **Descriptive:** Examination of subjects regarding a specific issue without a control group or randomization

Source: Flaugher, M. (2008). Nursing Research Program Builder: Strategies to Translate Findings into Practice. *Marblehead, MA: HCPro, Inc.*

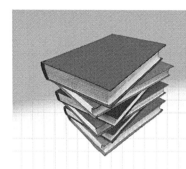

References

Aiken, L. (2002). Superior outcomes for Magnet hospitals. The evidence base. In M. McClure and A. Hinshaw (Eds.), *Magnet Hospitals Revisited: Attraction and Retention of Registered Nurses* (pp. 61–82). Washington, DC: American Nurses Publishing.

American Nurses Association. (2000). *Nurse Staffing and Patient Outcomes in the Inpatient Hospital Setting.* Washington, DC: American Nurses Association.

American Nurses Credentialing Center. (2004). *Application Manual for the Magnet Recognition Program®.* Silver Spring, MD: American Nurses Credentialing Center.

American Nurses Credentialing Center. (2009). Evidence based practice: Creating a culture of inquiry. Retrieved March 9, 2009, from *www.nursecredentialing.org/ Magnet/MagnetEvents/Magnet-Events-List/RecognitionWorkshops/EBP.aspx.*

Belcher, J. V. R., and Vonderhaar, K.J. (2005). Web-delivered research-based nursing staff education for seeking Magnet status. *Journal of Nursing Administration* 35 (9): 382–386.

Beyea, S. C. (2000). Getting started in nursing research and tips for success. *AORN Journal* 72 (6): 1061–1062.

Beyea, S.C., and Nicoll, L.H. (1997). Ten questions that will get you through any research report. *AORN Journal* 65 (5): 978–979.

Blegen, M., Goode, C., and Reed, L. (1998). Nursing staffing and patient outcomes. *Nursing Research* 47 (1): 43–50.

Brown, S. J. (1999). *Knowledge for Health Care Practice: A Guide to Using Research Evidence.* Philadelphia: W.B. Saunders.

Brown, S. J. (1999). Appraising findings from single original studies. In *Knowledge for Health Care Practice: A Guide to Using Research Evidence,* pp. 98–124. Philadelphia: W.B. Saunders.

Carper, B.A. (1988). Response to perspectives on knowing: A model of nursing knowledge. *Scholarly Inquiry for Nursing Practice* 2 (2): 141–144.

Clifford, C., and Murray, S. (2001). Pre- and post-test evaluation of a project to facilitate research development in practice in a hospital setting. *Journal of Advanced Nursing* 36 (5): 685–695.

Dontje, K.J. (2007). Evidence-based practice: Understanding the process. *Topics in Advanced Practice Nursing eJournal* 7(4). Retrieved March 9, 2009, from *www.medscape.com/viewarticle/567786.*

Dycoff, D. (2004). Doing it better: Improving practice with a journal club. *Nursing* 34 (7): 29.

ECRI Institute. (2009). Suggested guidelines for blood warmer use. Retrieved March 9, 2009, from *www.mdsr.ecri.org/summary/detail.aspx?doc_id=8269.*

Funk, S. G., Champagne, M.T., Wiese, R.A., and Tornquist, E.M. (1991). Barriers to using research findings in practice: the clinician's perspective. *Applied Nursing Research* 4 (2): 90–95.

Goode, C. J., and Piedalae, F. (1999). Evidence-based clinical practice. *Journal of Nursing Administration* 29 (6): 15–21.

Grinspun, D., Virani, T., and Bajnok, I. (2001/2002). Nursing best practice guidelines: The RNAO project. *Hospital Quarterly* 54–58.

Klapper, S. (2001). A tool to educate, critique, and improve practice. *AORN Journal* 74 (5): 712, 714–715.

Madsen, D., Sebolt, T., Cullen, L., Folkedahl, B., Mueller, T., Richardson, C., et al. (2005). Listening to bowel sounds: An evidence-based practice project. *American Journal of Nursing* 105 (12): 40–49.

Mateo, M.A., and Kirchhoff, K.T. (1999). *Using and Conducting Nursing Research in the Clinical Setting.* Philadelphia: W.B. Saunders Company.

McClure, M., and Hinshaw, A., (Eds.). (2002). *Magnet Hospitals Revisited: Attraction and Retention of Professional Nurses.* Washington, DC: American Nurses Publishing.

Moran-Peters, J. (2008). Positive effect of evidence-based nursing strategies on patient outcomes. Huntington Hospital Center for Nursing. Retrieved March 9, 2009 from *www.acestar.uthscsa.edu/institute/su08/documents/52Moran-Peters.pdf.*

Needleman, J., Bauerhouse, P., Mattke, S., Stewart, M., and Jalevinsky, K. (2002). Nurse staffing levels and the quality of care in hospitals. *The New England Journal of Medicine* 346 (22): 1715–1722.

Newhouse, R., Dearholt, S., Poe, S., Pugh, L.C., and White, K.M. (2005). Evidence-based practice: a practical approach to implementation. *Journal of Nursing Administration* 35 (1): 35–40.

Nicoll, L.H., and Beyea, S.C. (2000). Working with staff around evidence-based practice: The next generation of research utilization. *Seminars in Perioperative Nursing* 9: 133–142.

Pasek, T., and Zack, J. (2004). Cultivating a research milieu: Journal clubs in the pediatric intensive care unit. *Critical Care Nurse* 24 (6): 96–97.

Phillips, R., and Glasziou, P. (2004). What makes evidence-based journal clubs succeed? ACP Journal Club, 140, A11–A12. Retrieved January 9, 2006, from *www.acpjc.org/Content/140/3/issueACPJC-2004-140-3-A11.htm.*

Pravikoff, D.S., Tanner, A.B., and Pierce, S.T. (2005). Readiness of U. S. nurses for evidence-based practice. *American Journal of Nursing* 105 (9): 40–51.

Rosswurm, M.A., and Larrabee, J.H. (1999). A model to change to evidence-based practice. *Image: Journal of Nursing Scholarship.*

Sackett, D.L., et al. (1996). Evidence-based medicine: What it is and what it isn't. *British Medical Journal* 312: 71–72.

Scott, J., Sochalski, J., and Aiken, L. (1999). Review of the Magnet hospital research: Findings and implications for professional nursing practice. *Journal of Nursing Administration* 29 (1): 9–19.

Speers, A.T. (1999). An introduction to nursing research through an OR nursing journal club. *AORN Journal* 1232: 1235–1236.

Stevens, K.R. (2004). ACE Star Model of EBP: Knowledge Transformation. Academic Center for Evidence-based Practice. The University of Texas Health Science Center at San Antonio. Retrieved March 9, 2009, from *www.acestar. uthscsa.edu.*

Titler, M.G., Mentes, J., Rakel, B., Abbott, L., and Baumler, S. (1999). From Book
to Beside: Putting Evidence to Use in the Care of the Elderly. *Journal on Quality
Improvement:* 25(10): 545–556.

Titler, M.G., Kleiber, C., Steelman, V.J., Rakel, B.A., Budreau, G., Everett, L.Q., et
al. (2001). The Iowa model of evidence-based practice to promote quality care.
Critical Care Nursing Clinical of North America 13 (4): 497–509.

West, S., King, V., Carey, T. S., et al. (2002). Systems to rate the strength of
scientific evidence. Evidence Report/Technology Assessment No. 47. *AHRQ
Publication No. 02-E016.*

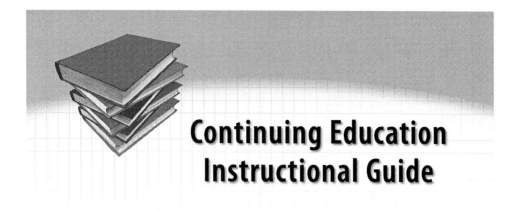

Continuing Education Instructional Guide

Quick-E! Pro: Evidence-Based Practice: A Guide for Nurses

Target Audience

Staff nurses

Charge nurses

Staff educators

Staff development specialists

Directors of education

Nurse managers

Statement of Need

A guide to help nurses understand evidence-based practice (EBP) and how they can conduct EBP projects. It walks readers through finding and using sources of evidence and guides them in conducting literature reviews. Implementing a culture of EBP will help nurses improve quality of care while boosting professional development and staff satisfaction. (This activity is intended for individual use only.)

Educational Objectives

Upon completion of this activity, participants should be able to:

■ Explain EBP

- Describe how EBP contributes to improved patient outcomes

- Discuss the resources needed for conducting EBP projects

- Examine strategies for creating a culture of EBP

- Identify various models of EBP

- Examine how models help structure EBP

- Discuss ways to get started with asking a question

- Discuss best practices for finding evidence

- Describe how to conduct a literature critique

- List online sources for evidence

- Evaluate various online sources of evidence

- Discuss best practices for sharing EBP information

Faculty

Joan Monchak Lorenz, MSN, RN, PMHCNS-BC, has a varied and well-rounded nursing career in clinical work, consultation and counseling, teaching, and research. She is a clinical nurse educator in the nursing education department at Bay Pines (FL) VA Healthcare System. In this capacity, she works on hospitalwide educational initiatives, provides unit-based programming, and consults with nursing staff on their professional growth. She supports evidence-based practice through her work on the Standards of Care Committee, as past chair of the Evidence-Based Practice Committee, and as past Coordinator of Evidence-Based Practice at Bay Pines.

Suzanne C. Beyea, RN, PhD, FAAN, is the director of nursing research at the Dartmouth-Hitchcock Medical Center (DHMC) in Lebanon, NH. Her responsibilities include supporting EBP, developing the clinical nursing research program for the medical center, and supporting nurses' efforts to use or conduct research. Her activities include providing consultation, education, technical support, and advice related to research, EBP, and the evaluation of nursing practices and clinical processes.

Mary Jo Slattery, RN, MS, is the nursing research coordinator at DHMC. She collaborates with the director of nursing research in the Office of Professional Nursing to support and facilitate research and EBP efforts in nursing. Her activities include consulting for and assisting groups and individuals on such topics as online searching, project planning, instrument development, obtaining Institutional Review Board (IRB) approval, data collection, data analysis, and report writing. She manages the departmental review for nursing research studies prior to submission to the IRB, coordinates the use of statistical analysis software, and conducts analysis on selected projects.

Nursing Contact Hours

HCPro, Inc., is accredited as a provider of continuing nursing education by the American Nurses Credentialing Center Commission on Accreditation.

This educational activity for 3 nursing contact hours is provided by HCPro, Inc.

Disclosure Statements

HCPro, Inc., has confirmed that none of the faculty or contributors have any relevant financial relationships to disclose related to the content of this educational activity.

Instructions

To be eligible to receive your nursing contact hours or physician continuing education credits for this activity, you are required to do the following:

1. Read the book *Quick-E! Pro: Evidence-Based Practice: A Guide for Nurses*

2. Complete the exam and receive a passing score of 80%

3. Complete the evaluation

4. Provide your contact information on the exam and evaluation

5. Submit exam and evaluation to HCPro, Inc.

Please provide all of the information requested above and mail or fax your completed exam, program evaluation, and contact information to:

> HCPro, Inc.
> Attention: Continuing Education Manager
> P.O. Box 1168
> Marblehead, MA 01945
> Fax: 781/639-2982

NOTE:

This book and associated exam are intended for individual use only. If you would like to provide this continuing education exam to other members of your nursing or physician staff, please contact our customer service department at 877/727-1728 to place your order. The exam fee schedule is as follows:

Exam Quantity	Fee
1	$0
2–25	$15 per person
26–50	$12 per person
51–100	$8 per person
101+	$5 per person

Continuing Education Exam

Name: _____

Title: _____

Facility name: _____

Address: _____

Address: _____

City: _____ State: _____ ZIP: _____

Phone number: _____ Fax number: _____

E-mail: _____

Date completed: _____

1. **Evidence-based practice (EBP) is the application of _____ to practice.**

    a. instinct

    b. tradition

    c. advice

    d. research

2. **Why might nurses who use EBP contribute to more improved patient outcomes than those who provide care in accordance to what they learned in nursing school?**

    a. EBP closes the gaps of an insufficient nursing education

    b. EBP eliminates nurses' risk of making a medical error

    c. EBP provides a critical strategy to ensure that care is up to date and reflects the latest research evidence

    d. EBP provides structure so that nurses deliver more competent care

3. **Which of the following statements best describes an EBP goal?**

    a. Achieve excellence in care delivery, even exceeding quality assurance standards

    b. Achieve excellence in care delivery by conducting nursing research

    c. Achieve excellence in care delivery by following nursing instincts

    d. Achieve excellence in care delivery by following standard nursing practice

4. **Which of the following is NOT needed to fully integrate EBP into an organization and ensure all nursing practice is based on evidence?**

    a. Accessible research reports and articles

    b. Administrative support

    c. Large nursing staff

    d. Knowledgeable mentors

5. **EBP projects rarely occur without the combined expertise of a group of clinicians who can:**

    a. Devote the majority of their time to them

    b. Undergo extensive training about EBP

    c. Collaborate frequently and effectively

    d. Readily access literature and have time to work on a specific project

6. **What strategy can nurses use to incorporate EBP concepts into nursing practice committees?**

    a. Informing experienced managers about the benefits EBP can have on patient care

    b. Educating peers about the importance and relevance of EBP in nursing

    c. Asking the chair of the nursing committee about the use of EBP when reviewing existing standards of nursing practice or implementing new ones

    d. Asking peers if they understand the meaning of EBP

7. **What might be one of the first steps to developing an EBP culture?**

    a. Conducting research for EBP projects

    b. Assessing the accessibility of electronic resources and computers and developing a plan to get needed resources

    c. Brainstorming topics for EBP projects

    d. Achieving leadership buy-in

8. **How can journal clubs be useful tools for creating a culture of EBP in nursing?**

    a. They provide nurses the opportunity to learn and develop skills to read and critically evaluate current research to determine how applicable the findings in their practice area are

    b. They offer nurses time to relieve stress surrounding patient care decisions

    c. They allow nurses the chance to build relationships to enhance collaborative practice

    d. They grant nurses the opportunity to communicate frequently and openly

9. **_____ was developed to describe knowledge transformation and to guide implementation of research into clinical practice considering the entire healthcare system, including the provider, the patient, and the infrastructure.**

    a. The Academic Center for Evidence-Based Nursing Star Model of Knowledge Transformation®

    b. The Iowa Model of EBP

    c. Rosswurm and Larrabee's Model for Change to Evidence-Based Practice

    d. The University of Colorado's Evidence-Based Multidisciplinary Clinical Practice Model

10. The Star Model of Knowledge Transformation® is a model for understanding the
_____, nature, and characteristics of knowledge that are used in various
aspects of EBP.

    a. phases

    b. traits

    c. qualities

    d. cycles

11. During the _____ stage of the Star Model of Knowledge Transformation®,
evidence summaries are transformed into practice recommendations and then
integrated into nursing practice.

    a. translation

    b. alteration

    c. changing

    d. transformation

12. Getting started in EBP requires nurses to identify problems, areas of concern,
and/or a:

    a. Source for information, such as a research article or journal

    b. Leader for driving EBP initiatives

    c. EBP project topic

    d. Clinical question

13. It is important that nurses focus their EBP question by:

    a. Developing one method that all nurses will agree to use

    b. Developing several methods that nurses will agree to use interchangeably

    c. Creating handout packets that will thoroughly explain the question

    d. Conducting a presentation that explains the aim of the question

14. **How does the PICO method assist nurses in structuring EBP?**

    a. It increases healthcare professionals' awareness in increasing patient safety

    b. It clarifies the physician's role in improving patient outcomes

    c. It helps nurses ask broad clinical questions

    d. It helps nurses ask pertinent clinical questions and focus on asking the right question

15. **In reference to "P" of the PICO model, nurses can focus their EBP question by identifying the _____.**

    a. patient's date of birth

    b. problem

    c. patient population

    d. patient outcome desired

16. **Which of the following are best practices nurses can use to find evidence?**

    a. Bulletin board Web sites

    b. Personal Web sites

    c. Adhering to methods peers use when conducting research

    d. Asking a librarian or an educator to come to an EBP council meeting to explain how to conduct literature searches

17. **When conducting a literature critique, nurses should organize their findings so they:**

    a. Can quickly identify any current information

    b. Can easily compare and contrast the conclusions or recommendations from the articles

    c. Avoid clutter during the research process

    d. Highlight the least important information

18. **Which of the following online sources are recommended as reputable professional healthcare Web sites nurses can access for evidence?**

    a. Yahoo

    b. Google

    c. Netting the Research

    d. The National Library of Medicine

19. **The Cochrane Library is an online resource for organized reports on EBP that reflect the best available information about:**

    a. Healthcare interventions and their effectiveness

    b. Healthcare interventions

    c. Healthcare education

    d. Healthcare planning

20. **What method can nurses use to share EBP information creatively with nurse colleagues about work related to EBP projects?**

    a. Disclosing information at staff meetings

    b. Conducting informational lectures

    c. EBP games, such as a crossword puzzle or bingo, to encourage participation, with small prizes, candy, or handouts as incentives

    d. Distributing informational handouts